How To Beat Insomnia And Sleepless

326 Effective Tips To Avoid Insomnia And Get A Good Night's Sleep

ADAM COLTON

Published by BizMove
www.bizmove.com

Table of Contents

1. Insomnia Fact Sheet

Insomnia is trouble falling asleep, staying asleep through the night, or waking up too early in the morning.

Episodes of insomnia may come and go or be long-lasting.

The quality of your sleep is as important as how much sleep you get.

Causes

Sleep habits we learned as children may affect our sleep behaviors as adults. Poor sleep or lifestyle habits that may cause insomnia or make it worse include:

- Going to bed at a different time each night
- Daytime napping
- Poor sleeping environment, such as too much noise or light
- Spending too much time in bed while awake
- Working evenings or night shifts
- Not getting enough exercise

- Using the television, computer, or a mobile device in bed

The use of some medicines and drugs may also affect sleep, including:

- Alcohol or other drugs
- Heavy smoking
- Too much caffeine throughout the day or drinking caffeine late in the day
- Getting used to certain types of sleep medicines
- Some cold medicines and diet pills
- Other medicines, herbs, or supplements

Physical, social, and mental health issues can affect sleep patterns, including:

- Bipolar disorder.
- Feeling sad or depressed. (Often, insomnia is the symptom that causes people with depression to seek medical help.)
- Stress and anxiety, whether it is short-term or long-term. For some people, the stress caused by insomnia makes it even harder to fall asleep.

Health problems may also lead to problems sleeping and insomnia:

- Pregnancy
- Physical pain or discomfort.

- Waking up at night to use the bathroom, common in men with enlarged prostate
- Sleep apnea

With age, sleep patterns tend to change. Many people find that aging causes them to have a harder time falling asleep, and that they wake up more often.

Symptoms

The most common complaints or symptoms in people with insomnia are:

- Trouble falling asleep on most nights
- Feeling tired during the day or falling asleep during the day
- Not feeling refreshed when you wake up
- Waking up several times during sleep

People who have insomnia are sometimes consumed by the thought of getting enough sleep. But the more they try to sleep, the more frustrated and upset they get, and the harder sleep becomes.

Lack of restful sleep can:

- Make you tired and unfocused, so it is hard to do daily activities.

- Put you at risk for auto accidents. If you are driving and feel sleepy, pull over and take a break.

Exams and Tests

Your health care provider will do a physical exam and ask about your current medications, drug use, and medical history. Usually, these are the only methods needed to diagnose insomnia.

Treatment

Not getting 8 hours of sleep every night does not mean your health is at risk. Different people have different sleep needs. Some people do fine on 6 hours of sleep a night. Others only do well if they get 10 to 11 hours of sleep a night.

Treatment often begins by reviewing any drugs or health problems that may be causing or worsen insomnia, such as:

- Enlarged prostate gland, causing men to wake up at night
- Pain or discomfort from muscle, joint, or nerve disorders

You should also think about lifestyle and sleep habits that may affect your sleep. This is called sleep hygiene. Making some changes in your sleep habits may improve or solve your insomnia.

Some people may need medicines to help with sleep for a short period of time. But in the long run, making changes in your lifestyle and sleep habits is the best treatment for problems with falling and staying asleep.

- Most over-the-counter (OTC) sleeping pills contain antihistamines. These medicines are commonly used to treat allergies. Your body quickly becomes used to them.
- Sleep medicines called hypnotics can be prescribed by your provider to help reduce the time it takes you to fall asleep. Most of these can become habit-forming.
- Medicines used to treat anxiety or depression can also help with sleep

Different methods of talk therapy may help you gain control over anxiety or depression.

Outlook (Prognosis)

Most people are able to sleep by practicing good sleep hygiene.

When to Contact a Medical Professional

Call your provider if insomnia has become a problem.

2. 326 Effective Tips To Avoid Insomnia And Get A Good Night's Sleep

People have been struggling with insomnia for a long time. It's something that can be caused by a number of things, and it's something that isn't just going to go away. If you'd like help in figuring out what you can do to treat your symptoms, then keep reading this book.

1. Avoid alcohol, caffeine, sugar and nicotine. These stimulants may be effective in keeping you awake during the day but they are also making it difficult for you to sleep at night. Limit their consumption throughout the day. Do not take any stimulants at least four hours before going to bed for the night.

2. Get used to sleeping on your back. Of all the sleeping positions, sleeping on your back causes the least stress on your internal organs while resting. This should help your entire body to relax enough to break insomnia. If back sleeping is not an option, the next best is sleeping on your right side.

3. Get in the habit of not sleeping in, even on the weekends. Sleeping for longer periods of time than you are used to can throw your entire sleep schedule out the door. For people that experience insomnia, this can kick it into high gear. Instead, set the alarm for the same time that you need to get up for on the weekdays.

4. Try using earplugs. It's often the sounds around the home or outside that are causing insomnia. So the best thing that you can do is stop yourself from hearing them. You can't stop traffic or birds, but you can block your ear canals with plugs. It may be just the silence you need.

5. Many people suffer from a racing mind as they try to fall asleep. This can keep you awake, distracting you from a restful night of sleep. For those who are not able to calm their thoughts, their minds need to be distracted. Putting on some white noise like the soft sound of a fan or rain can help keep your mind off of other things that may be keeping you awake.

6. Don't snack before bedtime. The sugar rush you experience will keep you awake. Not only that, but you'll find you're more likely to put on weight if you eat before bed. If you insist on

having something before you go to bed, try a bit of warm milk or some turkey.

7. Taking two tylenol when you go to sleep has always been a big tip for people with insomnia. However, you can trade this out with an ibuprofen. Or, you can substitute taking tylenol or ibuprofen with all-natural melatonin. All three of these are able to put you in a relaxed state.

8. You're probably not going to solve all of your problems while you're in bed. If you find yourself worrying about everything that could go wrong or problems that you need to solve, redirect your thoughts. Breath deeply and think about something relaxing or pleasant. If necessary, get up and write down the things that are keeping you from sleeping well.

9. Do not nap. While you may feel that you desperately need the rest, napping will keep you up later in the evenings. That means you'll just be tired again when you wake up, starting the whole cycle all over again. Keep yourself up during the day and you'll find that you are ready to sleep when your bedtime rolls around.

10. If your bedroom is not dark, it could be the reason why you have insomnia. Even the

smallest light can hinder many people from falling asleep. If your clock is too bright, buy a new one that only lights up when you press a button. If there is too much outside light, buy darkening curtains to help keep your bedroom dark.

11. If you find you wake up short of breath or in a panic, talk to your doctor about attending a sleep clinic. It is possible that you have sleep apnea, a condition where your airflow is cut off during the night. There are simple solutions for this condition which can give you the sleep you deserve.

12. Therapists are known to use imagery to help insomnia sufferers relax at night. Try lying in bed, lights off and no noise. Imagine yourself in the most peaceful place you can imagine, such as a beach with lapping waves, a rainforest with trickling rain or in a boat on a sunny lake. Imagery can help you fall asleep.

13. Being hungry before bed can cause you to not sleep well. You don't want to eat too much, but a small healthy snack can be enough to hold you over until the morning.

14. Of course you are tired through the day. You do not get enough sleep at night. You should avoid taking naps during the day. As hard as it may seem, it will make sleeping through the night even more difficult. When feeling tired during the day, go for a walk or do some aerobic exercises to wake yourself back up.

15. Try aromatherapy to help relax your mind and sooth your nerves. You can use a calming lavender bubble bath to relax in the tub. You might find that using a lavender scented laundry softener on your sheets works well too. Vanilla is also relaxing so consider using vanilla if you don't like lavender.

16. Magnesium is one mineral that has been shown to help people fall asleep. If you are not keen on taking it as a supplement, you can take a bath in it. A warm bath with a few handfuls of Epsom salt will help you get to sleep a lot faster.

17. Only sleep enough to be refreshed the next day. Too much sleep can actually help create insomnia the next evening. And not enough sleep can stress the body out in ways that also trigger insomnia. Try to get just enough rest - somewhere between 7 and 9 hours at maximum.

18. Talk with your doctor if you are experiencing insomnia. While insomnia may just be cause by things like stress and anxiety, it can also be a symptom of certain physical disorders. Don't self diagnose. Speak with your general practitioner immediately. The doctor will be able to tell you what the cause is and give you the proper treatment.

19. Play some music right before you go to bed. Music can have a really relaxing effect on the body, and that's important for those suffering from insomnia. Choose music that calms you, and have it playing lightly in the background as you lay down for sleep. Don't go with any music that's energizing. That's the wrong direction you want to go!

20. If you're experiencing insomnia for over 30 minutes, get up. Staying in bed may worsen the situation. Rather, do something that's quiet, relaxing, and offers little stimulation. When you start feeling tired again, try going back to bed and see what happens. You may need to do this multiple times in a night.

21. Don't do other things in your bed, other than sleep. This means no television watching, reading, or doing any sort of puzzles before bed.

All of these things can stimulate your brain, and that can trigger insomnia. When sleeping is the sole function of the bed, you'll be more likely to get the rest you need.

22. If sleep absolutely eludes you, do not just lie there worrying about sleeping. Try getting out of bed, and doing some light activity, such as a warm bath, or a little reading. This may be just enough activity to make you forget about your sleep problems, and help you to fall asleep.

23. If you've tried everything else for your insomnia, why not consider self-hypnosis? Talking yourself into a state of sleepiness can mean falling asleep much faster. You could also play recordings of a hypnotist which are geared to this purpose. The repetitive words in a calm voice should help you work around the insomnia.

24. Practice breathing deeply when you are in bed. Breathing deeply can really relax your entire body. This will aid in the sleep process. Breathe long inhales and exhales, repeatedly. Breathe in with your nose and out with your mouth. You might even be ready for sleep in as little as a few minutes.

25. It's hard to sleep when you aren't actually tired. If you have a job that requires you to be sedentary, take frequent breaks and move around throughout the day. Exercise is a great way to get in physical exercise that helps you sleep at bedtime.

26. Your problem may actually lie with your bed. If your mattress is too hard, you may find it next to impossible to get into a comfortable sleeping position. The same goes for a bed which is too soft, or even pillows which aren't the right height or hardness for you.

27. Cut down on fluid intake before you go to sleep. If you have to wake up in the middle of your sleep to go to the bathroom, you have to make sure that you cut the fluids you have in the evening so you can have uninterrupted sleep instead of getting up over and over.

28. Don't use your bedroom for anything except sleeping and dressing. Fighting, using a computer, or the like can make your brain view the room as the place for those activities to occur. You'll be able to train your brain into thinking your bedroom is for sleep, if that's the only thing you do there.

29. Creating a proper sleep environment is essential. Look around and eliminate the things that bother you and keep you from sleep. Block off sources of light that can't be turned off. If you can't eliminate an annoying sound, the try using a white noise to cover it and to allow yourself to drift off.

30. Take a bath that is warm, almost hot. In addition, add some Epsom salt or baking soda. That will make you feel calmer. The salts can soothe your muscles, and you might be more likely to fall asleep when you make an attempt later in the evening. Don't make it too hot or too cold.

31. Think about the things that bother you as you toss and turn. Now do something about them before you go to bed. Block out annoying lights and noises. Set the temperature at a cooler setting so you aren't hot and kicking off covers.If you eliminate the things that keep you awake, then sleep should come much easier.

32. If you want to fall asleep easier, it is best to go to bed when you are feeling particularly sleepy. Trying to force yourself to sleep at a predetermined time is not going to help. Since

you are not tired at this time, you will only end up laying there restlessly.

33. Stop lying in bed worrying about not sleeping. Should you find yourself unable to fall asleep, target an activity that will get it off your mind. For some people it might be reading or writing, for others, it may involve getting out of bed and going for a walk. Do not be afraid to do something to help, as opposed to lying about worrying when sleep will come.

34. Try to keep things that are distracting out of the bedroom area. This only makes it more difficult for you to get to sleep. This means that computers, televisions and other electronics should not be in there. If they must be there, turn them off as soon as you are ready to hit the sheets.

35. Talk with your doctor if you are experiencing insomnia. While insomnia may just be cause by things like stress and anxiety, it can also be a symptom of certain physical disorders. Don't self diagnose. Speak with your general practitioner immediately. The doctor will be able to tell you what the cause is and give you the proper treatment.

36. Many folks like to be night owls on holidays and weekends. However, not sleeping at the same time every night can make insomnia occur. Set an alarm to make yourself awaken the same time every day. After a few days, you will develop a sleep routine.

37. Try not to take naps. Napping can interrupt the normal sleep schedule, making it harder to fall asleep at bedtime. Try to associate sleep with darkness and relaxation. You will be more likely to fall asleep easily if you are tired from being awake all day, instead of feeling refreshed from an earlier nap.

38. If your doctor prescribes sleeping medication, take it exactly as the label says. Sleep medicine should be taken right before bedtime because they are designed to act quickly. Never drive after taking a sleeping pill. Never drink alcohol while taking sleeping pills. If you decide to quit taking your medication, talk to your doctor first.

39. See a doctor. You might not be able to find your insomnia on your own, and you might need a professional to help. A doctor can make sure that there is not some other underlying condition causing you to miss sleep. He can also help you to try some sleep medication if necessary.

40. Try deep rhythmic breathing to snap out of a bout with insomnia. Lay in bed with your eyes closed and simply breathe with deliberation. This exercise will relax you and help take the focus off of the price you will pay tomorrow for not getting enough sleep tonight. Try counting the breaths too, to get sleepy faster.

41. Your pituitary gland produces melatonin which helps regulate your sleep. When the pituitary gland does not receive enough sunlight to produce vitamin D, you will have trouble falling asleep at night. Try to get about 10 or 15 minutes of sun every day so that your pituitary gland can work properly and help you fall asleep.

42. Visit your doctor if you are suffering from insomnia. Many times insomnia is only temporary; however, there may be an underlying medical problem causing your insomnia. Talk to a doctor to make sure nothing serious is wrong.

43. Stay away from alcohol. A lot of people try to soothe their sleep issues with alcohol, but that is not a good idea. For one thing, you don't want to become dependent on alcohol. For another thing, alcohol is a diuretic and may encourage

nighttime urination and difficulty when you want to go back to sleep.

44. Have a massage done. It doesn't have to be a professional; it can be your spouse. Just make sure they apply the strokes that are characteristic of a good massage. A nice massage can relax your muscles and put you into a relaxed state. That can make you more likely to sleep.

45. Try taking a relaxing trip to the mountains to help promote sleep. Daily activities in the mountains such biking and hiking will help you with the needed exercise. Sleeping in a tent will let you experience your life through new eyes and provide you with fresh air that can help you fall asleep.

46. Turn your bedroom into the perfect sleep environment. Block out all light, including the little LEDs which seem to be on everything. A small square of black electrical tape can do the trick. Next, block out noise or cover it up with a running fan or white noise machine.

47. The ideal temperature for your room when sleeping is slightly colder at 60-65 degrees. Why? This helps you relax, while warmer temperatures will cause you to toss and turn. So, instead of

adjusting the temperature away from this number, add or remove blankets accordingly. This helps you be able to get comfortable and get to sleep.

48. Of course you are tired through the day. You do not get enough sleep at night. You should avoid taking naps during the day. As hard as it may seem, it will make sleeping through the night even more difficult. When feeling tired during the day, go for a walk or do some aerobic exercises to wake yourself back up.

49. So, you go to bed and lie there waiting to go to sleep. If you are not having any success in falling asleep, get out of bed and wait a while. Read a book or watch some TV until you begin to feel your eyes getting heavy. It will make you feel much better if you go to bed when you are actually tired.

50. Don't let your clock stare at you and keep you awake. Turn it away from you. While you may not think it is a big deal, it can cause huge distractions for some people. You can keep the clock near by, but turn the face away from you.

51. There are people who deal with insomnia that understand how to fool their mind into getting

sleepy. Imagine that it is morning time. They visualize their alarm going off. If you can focus your mind on that feeling of wanting to shut off the alarm, you might be able to trick your mind into falling back asleep.

52. You can invite sleep in by creating a dark, soothing atmosphere in your bedroom. Be sure to get shades or curtains that block any outside light. Try some soothing music, or a CD with ocean or bird sound effects. Read a relaxing book. Find what works for you, and create a habit of it. You will learn to associate these activities with sleep.

53. Have a bedtime ritual. Let your body know that sleeping is coming by doing the same things every night. For example, you might try having a hot bath, hot tea and reading in bed for about half an hour. This practice will be more effective if you are consistent, so keep it up.

54. Regular exercise can help to curb insomnia. A good workout can tire you out, and get you ready for sleep. However, exercising too close to bedtime can be a stimulant, making your insomnia worse. Be sure to stop exercising at least three hours before bedtime to avoid aggravating insomnia.

55. For people who have trouble falling asleep at night, many herbs have been used to help people sleep for centuries. Some herbs that are helpful in inducing sleep are passionflower or chamomile tea, California poppy, kava, valerian and hops. These herbs will relax the body and help induce restful sleep.

56. Create a diary with your sleep patterns to find any problems that you could be having. Jot down what you have eaten before bed, your exercise habits as well as your moods each day. See if this helps you to get more sleep. By understanding what factors help you get more or less rest, you can make necessary changes.

57. Smoking is not good for you in so many ways, including helping to cause insomnia. Your heart rate goes up and your body is stimulated, too. There are so many reasons why you should quit smoking. Improving the quality of your sleep is just one of many benefits.

58. If you are having trouble sleeping, have your doctor run some tests. A simple blood test can detect your levels of magnesium and calcium. Both of these minerals are important for sleep. Although you can take dietary supplements, it is

better if you can get an adequate amount of these minerals from dietary sources.

59. If you find you wake up shaking in the night, but a thick blanket doesn't help, have a glass of warm milk before you hit the hay. Milk contains nutrients which keep your blood sugar level overnight, and this can save you from that horrible shaking you are experiencing.

60. Try not to eat spicy foods for dinner or you may end up in discomfort at bedtime. Spicy foods can cause heartburn, and this can cause you to have problems falling or staying asleep. Keep the spice to lunch and you may find that you can sleep better at night.

61. If you find you are tired during the day, consider taking a ten minute nap in the afternoon. This can rejuvenate you just enough to give you energy, but it won't cause you to not be able to fall asleep at night. If you stick to a routine, that will help even more.

62. Many people drink alcohol a little while before bed because it has been known to make them a little drowsy. While this may be true, drinking alcohol also increases the chances of you waking

up several times over the course of the night without being able to fall back asleep.

63. Practicing deep breathing techniques will help you when you are having trouble sleeping. Lie on your back to relax. Take deep breaths, inhaling as much as you can, and pause for a few seconds before starting to exhale slowly. After around five or ten minutes of this, you will notice a pervasive sense of calm.

64. A little while before bedtime, eat a snack that is high in carbohydrates. At first, your blood sugar levels will be elevated. The insulin will kick in and your blood sugar level will fall causing you to get drowsy. This is a good way to begin your night's slumber.

65. Try aromatherapy to help relax your mind and sooth your nerves. You can use a calming lavender bubble bath to relax in the tub. You might find that using a lavender scented laundry softener on your sheets works well too. Vanilla is also relaxing so consider using vanilla if you don't like lavender.

66. If you are suffering from insomnia, one simple solution is sex. Not only does sex relieve tension, but it helps relax the body so that it can fall

asleep. It does not matter if you are alone or with others, having sex can provide the necessary stimulation and relaxation needed for you to fall asleep.

67. If you are exhausted and suffering from lack of sleep, an afternoon nap can seem very tempting. Nevertheless, napping during the day is not a good solution for insomnia. You need to work on developing regular sleep habits, and napping can disrupt your schedule. Daytime napping can actually sap the effectiveness of your nighttime sleep.

68. Although it a good idea to avoid food before you go to bed, some light snacks may promote sleep. Foods with carbohydrates and tryptophan can help you sleep better. Foods like turkey, whole grain cereal or a banana can help some people rest better. See if these foods work for you.

69. Don't read right before going to bed. You may love the time you have right before bed to get a few chapters in, but really you are stimulating your body. If you're battling insomnia that's the last thing that you want to do. So keep the books out of the room.

70. Stay away from anything that has caffeine in it. For example, you would not want to consume coffee or sugary soda just before going to bed. In addition, although herbal tea is recommended for sleep, black tea is not. If you get the two confused, you may find it even more difficult to fall asleep than before.

71. If OTC sleeping aids are something you are considering, make sure you get your doctor's blessing first. This is especially important if you are going to take it for an extended period of time. It might be safe for occasional use, but could pose problems on your body after extended use.

72. You should write your issues in a sleep diary. Jot down what you have eaten before bed, your exercise habits as well as your moods each day. Then look at the amount of rest you are getting. By understanding what factors help you get more or less rest, you can make necessary changes.

73. Even if you are very tired, resist the urge to sleep in on the weekends. If you let yourself rest for an extra hour or two, you could mess up your sleeping schedule for the week. Once you wake up, get out of bed. Do not allow yourself to fall back asleep or to stay in bed for a while.

74. Start regular exercise to combat insomnia. Many people face stress and tension throughout the day. Without a good release, these feelings can compound as bed time draws near. Set a regular schedule of walking, running or exercise for a short time each day, that can relieve these tensions and allow your mind and body to unwind properly.

75. Take notes on your nights to figure out what is keeping you awake. First, write in your journal what happened during the day. It is also helpful to keep a diet diary along with your journal as what you eat or drink may be affecting your sleep. Next, write how you feel in the morning. Review it to figure out the cause of your woes.

76. If you want to have a bedtime snack, do so at least an hour before bed. This gives your stomach time to process the food, ensuring that you don't feel full or bloated when you lie down. This can also help with the heartburn you may deal with at bed time.

77. Drink a delicious cup of herbal tea before bedtime. There are several teas on the market with herbs that are helpful in relaxing the body. You can try fennel, anise, cat nip or chamomile.

You can find these teas at many super markets or your local health food store.

78. To soothe your body, a hot cup of herbal, non-caffeinated tea might do the trick. Just drink one cup, though, otherwise you may find yourself getting up during the night to use the bathroom. Be sure that the tea contains no caffeine or it might be the culprit which keeps you awake!

79. Do not take naps if you you suffer from insomnia. Naps are darn tempting, but they can be counterproductive. Do what you can to get through your day awake at all times, and you are more likely to find sleep in the evening.

80. Amazingly enough, your sleep problems might be caused by not getting enough sunlight. A lack of sun exposure can cause your body to not produce the nutrients it needs for your brain to operate correctly. Get outside for at least 30 minutes a day to ensure you are able to sleep.

81. Don't get too worked up about having insomnia. When you find yourself lying in bed again unable to sleep, it's easy to start getting frustrated and impatient. However, that behavior is not going to help usher in sleep. Try to realize

that for many, insomnia can be fixed to some degree.

82. For your afternoon snack, avoid eating foods which are processed. Instead, eat some fresh fruit, yogurt or nuts. This will give you the energy boost you need without leaving you crashing or affected by high levels of sodium. Both situations can cause you to have trouble falling asleep at night.

83. There's nothing like a couple drinks to relax from a long, busy day. Next time you go to grab a beer, opt out, and if you must, be sure you are sobered up and hydrated before bed. Although alcohol can be a sedative and cause sleepiness, it is more likely to provide a less restful sleep.

84. Eating a bedtime snack can help you feel sedated. Try a piece of whole grain toast with some honey along with a glass of warm milk. This will fill you up, help you become drowsy and leave you ready to hit the sack. Enjoy it 2 hours before bed for the best results.

85. Don't think too much about sleep if you have trouble at night. While you do want to fall asleep if you suffer from insomnia, thinking about it too much can cause stress, making the problem

worse. Instead of thinking about sleep, think about steps to take to feel more relaxed. Then sleep will come naturally.

86. If you are suffering from long-term insomnia, consult your doctor. Ask if any of your regular medications could be interfering with your sleep schedule. Never take over-the-counter medications to help you sleep because you may become dependent on them. Your goal should be to fall asleep on your own every night.

87. When insomnia is the enemy, reserve the use of your bed for sleep only. Sleep experts say that using your bed for reading, writing or watching TV will devalue it as a sleep aid. If your mind sees your bed as a place for sleeping only, your body will be conditioned to fall asleep faster.

88. Don't do other things in your bed, other than sleep. This means no television watching, reading, or doing any sort of puzzles before bed. All of these things can stimulate your brain, and that can trigger insomnia. When sleeping is the sole function of the bed, you'll be more likely to get the rest you need.

89. You should think about giving your belly a rub. This will stimulate your stomach and aid you in

beating insomnia. This will help relax your body and improve digestion. If the responsible party for your insomnia is your stomach, this should do the trick.

90. For some, eating a small snack before bed can help them rest. Choose a food with both protein and carbohydrates. For example, both cookies and juice are options that would work. Consume the snack at least 45 minutes prior to laying down to bed and see if you are able to drift off sooner or easier than before.

91. Leave tablets and laptops in another room. It's tempting to bring your gadgets to bed, but they can easily keep you awake. Turn these devices off about an hour before bedtime for the best results. Let your body have the relax time that it needs.

92. Try finding a soothing and calming tea that you can sip on an hour or so before bed. Make sure it's an herbal tea that contains no caffeine at all. The best kinds for sleep would probably be chamomile or some kind of a mint tea. Experiment with the blends that say they're for sleeping as well.

93. Cognitive therapy can help you with your insomnia. This kind of therapy is going to help you figure out what you're doing wrong and how your thinking is affecting you when you're trying to sleep. Cognitive therapy also gives patients information so that they know exactly what they should be doing for their sleep routine.

94. A good massage prior to bedtime is helpful. It will calm your body and relax your muscles. In order to help your spouse sleep better as well, alternate nights giving the massage. It needn't be a marathon massage. Most people benefit from 15-minute hand, neck, or foot massages.

95. If your insomnia is very severe, talk to your doctor about prescription sleep medications. While these medications are useful in treating insomnia, they are not to be taken on a long-term basis, as they can aggravate insomnia in the long run. They are best used in order to establish a sleep routine, and are then discontinued.

96. Your bedroom should be an environment that is designed for restful sleep. It needs to be dark, quiet and comfortable. Keep it at a temperature that is not too cold or too hot. When you combine all these things together, your bedroom

will be the perfect environment to sleep in and you will not have trouble falling asleep.

97. Drink a warm glass of milk about 15 minutes before bedtime. Drinking warm milk is a great way to calm and soothe the nervous system. The calcium in the milk is what works in the nervous system to take the edge of and help you relax. When you are relaxed, you are more likely to fall asleep easier.

98. Many people suffer from insomnia because they cannot get their brain to shut down at night. One way to eliminate this is to write down any worries or problems before you go to bed. This will help your brain relax. When you make a list of your problems to be handled the next day, your brain can focus on what it needs to be doing, sleeping.

99. If your room temperature is far too warm, there is a chance that this will make it hard for you to sleep. While you want your room to be at a great comfort level, avoid cranking up the heat when it is time for bed. It should be at a neutral temperature and you can cozy under the blankets if you need more heat.

100. How much sleep you get will affect how much weight you lose. If you don't sleep enough, you'll be hungry all day. This also leads to poor decision-making on your part, whether at school, work, or home.

101. Use your bed for sleep and don't use it as a place for activities like watching television. Don't take your laptop to bed, and use it to finish work. You want the bed to be a relaxing place. You don't want it mentally tied to stressful activities that don't involve rest or love.

102. Don't drink a lot of liquids right before you go to bed. Doing so means you may wake up numerous times during the night, interrupting your valuable sleep. Drinks like tea and coffee are even worse. Not only do they contain caffeine, a mild stimulant that keeps you awake, they are a diuretic as well.

103. Avoid alcohol, caffeine, sugar and nicotine. These stimulants may be effective in keeping you awake during the day but they are also making it difficult for you to sleep at night. Limit their consumption throughout the day. Do not take any stimulants at least four hours before going to bed for the night.

104.   Find ways to deal with tension and stress. Starting your day with moderate exercise can help to ward off stress. Exercising strenuously before going to bed will keep you from getting your shuteye. Try practicing meditation or yoga right before you get in bed. Through these techniques, you can relax your overstimulated mind.

105.   Be sure to get ample physical exercise. People who have jobs that are physical are less troubled with insomnia than those who have an office job. You need to get your body tired out from time to time so it can rest better. Try walking for one or two miles when you return home after work.

106.   Don't do other things in your bed, other than sleep. This means no television watching, reading, or doing any sort of puzzles before bed. All of these things can stimulate your brain, and that can trigger insomnia. When sleeping is the sole function of the bed, you'll be more likely to get the rest you need.

107.   Don't automatically reach for prescription medicine when you can't fall asleep, as this can quickly become a dangerous habit. Insomnia is often temporary or simply due to something

stressful going on in your life. Try other things first, like warm milk or a bath, and make sure you get an okay from your doctor before trying the heavy stuff.

108.   Hot water bottles can help you sleep. This heat can relieve tension. It might be enough to let you fall asleep. One thing you can do is put a hot water bottle on your tummy. Breathe deeply and relax as the heat dissipates throughout your body.

109.   Read about the side effects and dangers of sleeping medications before deciding to take them. Sleeping pills can work short-term, but speak to a doctor before using them. Not just that, but you ought to read yourself and find out what risks there are.

110.   If you have trouble falling asleep at night, try keeping yourself on a regular sleep schedule. A regular sleep schedule is crucial if you are having trouble falling asleep. When you go to bed at about the same time on a daily basis, your body will be programmed to sleep better and fall asleep quicker.

111.   Introduce a nightly ritual of quiet time before bed. Television, smartphone and tablet

use are common for many people as they prepare to sleep. These devices can create over-stimulation in your brain and prevent the proper shutdown needed for rest. Avoid these devices and opt for a good book or writing in a journal.

112.   If you find you wake up short of breath or in a panic, talk to your doctor about attending a sleep clinic. It is possible that you have sleep apnea, a condition where your airflow is cut off during the night. There are simple solutions for this condition which can give you the sleep you deserve.

113.   Regular exercise is a great way to battle insomnia. This exercise will help relieve tension that is built up during the day and you should be able to fall asleep at night. Make sure that you do your exercise in the morning or during the day. Exercise before bedtime is not a good idea because it stimulates your body and wakes it up.

114.   Incorporate some carbohydrates in your dinner or nightly snack. Carbohydrates increase your blood sugar when eaten. However, when your body begins to produce insulin in response, this will elicit drowsiness. Do not over indulge with snacks though. Too much snack at night

can have the opposite effect. Keep it light and at a time that will give your body time to process it.

115.   Make sure the lights are dimmed when you try to sleep. This helps your body realize it is time for bed. You are going to start relaxing and getting drowsy, so that when the lights are fully off, you fall right asleep. Watching TV is counterproductive; the flickering screen has a sunrise effect. Shut off your TV at least two hours before going to bed.

116.   Do not spend your nights looking at the clock. You will drive yourself crazy. You likely need to have a clock in your room to help wake you in the morning, but that doesn't mean that you have to have it facing you. Turn the clock around so you do not see the time and you will be able to relax more and sleep better.

117.   One tip which can help you fall asleep is to immerse your senses in a single word. For example, begin by saying the word "sleep" in your head over and over again, slowly and softly. Then picture the word "sleep", then make it three dimensional. Try to hear a lullaby and feel your body falling asleep. Soon enough, you will be asleep!

118.   It has been shown that getting massages helps stimulate sleep, so ask someone for a rubdown when it is near your bedtime. Play soft music while getting this massage to further relax your brain. For extra effect, have you feet rubbed during this massage. There are acupressure points there that will stimulate sleep.

119.   Gently massage your abdomen. A tummy rub will stimulate your stomach and help fight off insomnia. Rubbing your tummy improves digestion and relaxes the body. If the responsible party for your insomnia is your stomach, this should do the trick.

120.   Do not keep your bedroom too hot. Keeping your sleeping area too warm can disturb sleep, and cause frequent waking. On the other hand, studies show no evidence that a cool room can cause sleep disturbances. Keeping the temperature low, and a window open may help to keep insomnia at bay.

121.   While often any distraction can disrupt sleeping, such as television or music, consider some soft classical music. Many people have claimed that playing some classical music while they're going to bed has helped them get some

sleep. It is this relaxed state that you may need to find sleep quickly.

122.   Blue light is known to suppress the production of melatonin, the hormone that helps you sleep. Be sure to avoid blue light from things like laptops, tvs, and phones for at least thirty minutes before bedtime. This will help your brain know it's power down time and not play time.

123.   If you suffer from insomnia frequently, try using aromatherapy to soothe you to sleep. Scented oils, such as lavender, are particularly relaxing, and are known to help with sleep. Try dabbing some on your pillow, or wearing some lavender body spray to bed. You can even make lavender sachets to keep on your night table.

124.   Caffeine can be a huge cause of insomnia. It stimulates your brain and metabolism, stopping your sleep. You may not realize just how early in the day you should stop consuming anything caffeinated. If you have insomnia, you should stop consuming caffeine at two o'clock in the afternoon.

125.   For the perfect pre-bed sedative, warm up a glass of milk and add a tablespoon of honey to it.

The combination of warm milk and sweet honey can help to sedate you very quickly. It also fills your tummy, plus milk has a long lasting effect on blood sugar, keeping you from having hunger pains overnight.

126.   Therapists are known to use imagery to help insomnia sufferers relax at night. Try lying in bed, lights off and no noise. Imagine yourself in the most peaceful place you can imagine, such as a beach with lapping waves, a rainforest with trickling rain or in a boat on a sunny lake. Imagery can help you fall asleep.

127.   If you get up at the same time every day, this will increase your chances of sleeping through the night. Since your body will become accustomed to sleeping for a certain number of hours, every time you go to bed you should sleep for the same number of hours each time.

128.   Try not to worry when you are going to sleep. This can lead to insomnia. If you are worrying about something, get up and do something relaxing until you feel like falling asleep again. If you lie in bed worrying about problems, that is all you will be able to do and not fall asleep.

129.   If you find yourself bored in the afternoon, go for a quick walk. That little bit of exercise can be enough to bring your energy levels up and allow you to be a little more tired at bed time. In the early evening, a walk after dinner can have the same results.

130.   Take a nice warm bath an hour before bedtime. Use lavender soap or body wash and light some scented candles. Use all of your senses to help you get tired. Once you get out of the bath, do not do anything that could arouse you so that you can easily fall into a deep slumber.

131.   If you find that the fear of your alarm going off keeps you up, or causes you to awaken and not be able to fall asleep, consider buying a different alarm clock. There are clocks which use the gradual addition of light to the room which wake you calmly and leave you well rested.

132.   If your partner keeps you awake all night, be honest with them. If they have restless legs and end up kicking you, let them know. If their snoring is driving you crazy, speak up. Obviously they're not getting a good sleep either, so guide them to their family doctor for help.

133.   If you find your bed isn't comfortable, invest in a new one. A mattress which is too firm or too soft can totally ruin your sleep. The same goes for your pillow, sheets and bed clothes. Invest in the best so that your sleep can be uninterrupted, providing you with the rest you need.

134.   Do not consume any spicy foods before you go to bed at night. Spicy foods can raise your blood pressure and increase your body temperature, which can have a very negative impact on the way that you feel before bed. Instead, drink water or eat an ice pop to appease your condition.

135.   Avoid each of the triggers of stress at night before you go to bed. Sometimes, an argument with someone that you love could cause you to become stressed three hours later when you have to go to bed. Make sure that you also get your work problems out of your head before bed.

136.   Stress is a major cause of many insomnia cases. So, in order to fight against insomnia, it's crucial to decrease your stress levels. Obviously, some stresses causes cannot be completely eliminated, so you need to know how to deal with it. Yoga and deep breathing can both be helpful with this.

137.   When your insomnia is getting the best of
        you, try a cup of warm milk. Although many
        people think this is just an old wives tale, there's
        really some science behind it. Warm milk actually
        soothes your nervous system, making sleep come
        more easily. Just pop a mug in the microwave for
        a minute or so and sleep should soon follow.

138.   If you can't sleep because you are worried
        about something in particular, get up and write it
        down. Sometimes putting your thoughts on
        paper will help ease your anxiety. You could also
        try to busy yourself with small but productive
        tasks that need to be done around the house. Go
        back to bed as soon as you begin to feel sleepy.

139.   Cut down on your caffeine intake. Caffeine
        can keep working for up to 24 hours, so if you
        are drinking a lot of coffee, that could be what is
        keeping you up. Try tapering off, and having a
        little less coffee every day. That way, you don't to
        quit caffeine cold turkey, which could result in
        withdrawal symptoms.

140.   Limit the amount of time you spend in bed.
        Your bed is for sleeping and not to pay your bills
        or make phone calls. It is also important that you
        refrain from listening to your radio or watching

your television while in bed. These types of activities make you alert and make it extra difficult to fall asleep.

141.   Do not nap. While you may feel that you desperately need the rest, napping will keep you up later in the evenings. That means you'll just be tired again when you wake up, starting the whole cycle all over again. Keep yourself up during the day and you'll find that you are ready to sleep when your bedtime rolls around.

142.   If you want to sedate yourself without taking sleeping pills and feeling like a zombie in the morning, try a cookie. Sugar eaten 30 minutes before bed time can actually cause you to become tired. You can also try honey in hot water or on a piece of toast for the same effect.

143.   Create a nightly routine and stick to it. It can be as simple as taking a warm bath, putting on comfortable sleep wear and reading a relaxing book. By developing a routine, you are conditioning your body to prepare for sleep. This can help you get into a comfortable rhythm of sleeping at the same time each night.

144.   If you get up at the same time every day, this will increase your chances of sleeping through

the night. Since your body will become accustomed to sleeping for a certain number of hours, every time you go to bed you should sleep for the same number of hours each time.

145.   Get some sun on your face. Sun in small doses is actually good for the body. Aim to get at least 15 minutes of sun on your face and you may find this helps you sleep better at night. The sun helps your body know it is daytime and this helps get your body into a sleep pattern.

146.   Of course you are tired through the day. You do not get enough sleep at night. You should avoid taking naps during the day. As hard as it may seem, it will make sleeping through the night even more difficult. When feeling tired during the day, go for a walk or do some aerobic exercises to wake yourself back up.

147.   Try aromatherapy to help relax your mind and sooth your nerves. You can use a calming lavender bubble bath to relax in the tub. You might find that using a lavender scented laundry softener on your sheets works well too. Vanilla is also relaxing so consider using vanilla if you don't like lavender.

148.   See if biofeedback works for you. You may consult a therapist for the initial session and then take the CDs home with you to listen to at night. Biofeedback helps you relax by focusing on each part of your body and releasing stress from it. It can be very effective if you are committed to it.

149.   Magnesium is one mineral that has been shown to help people fall asleep. If you are not keen on taking it as a supplement, you can take a bath in it. A warm bath with a few handfuls of Epsom salt will help you get to sleep a lot faster.

150.   Shift work can throw a monkey wrench into your normal sleep schedule. The human body is not designed to change it's sleep patterns every week. If possible, try to avoid switching shifts too often. Even if you have have to take a shift you don't like, try to keep to one shift as long as possible.

151.   There are many applications that help you fall asleep. Choose a sleep application that place relaxing white noise. Some of the options on the applications also record your sleep patterns so you can find the root cause of your sleep deprevation. There are many free applications available to help you sleep.

152. Sometimes a glass of wine as you relax in the evening can help you drift off to a peaceful sleep. It is mostly because the wine reduces any stress you are feeling, but it also makes some people feel drowsy. However, do not use alcohol to excess at any time.

153. If insomnia is a problem for you, see your doctor so any other medical conditions can be ruled out. There are many serious issues like clogged breathing and migraines that can cause serious insomnia. Treating these ailments can foster much better sleep.

154. Create a bedtime routine, and follow it faithfully each night. You could start by watching a favorite show with a cup of herbal tea. A bath, or washing your face, and flossing your teeth could come next. Get into bed, and read a peaceful book, or devotional, then turn the lights off. Once you get used to the routine, sleep should be the natural next step.

155. Rub your tummy to calm yourself down. Keeping your stomach stimulated is a great way to beat insomnia. You'll relax and your digestion will improve. If your stomach causes your insomnia, this is great techique to try first.

156.   Even though warm milk may help you fall asleep, some people do not like milk or cannot ingest dairy products. Try having some herbal tea. This tea has ingredients that will make you feel more relaxed. There are also special blends that can help you relax. Look to a health store to see what kind may work best for you.

157.   Stop taking naps. If you take a nap during the day, you are going to have a harder time going to sleep and staying asleep at night. When you cut out your nap, you will find that you have a better time remaining asleep when you go to sleep for the night.

158.   You may already know that regular exercise helps you get enough sleep, but it can also actually improve the quality of your sleep, too. However, it is important that you avoid exercising before your bedtime as it can act as a stimulant. Get your exercising over and done with a minimum of 3 hours prior to bedtime so that your sleep is not disrupted.

159.   While often any distraction can disrupt sleeping, such as television or music, consider some soft classical music. Some people claim it helps them sleep better. It can help your body calm down and find sleep.

160.   Try to reduce your stress before you're ready for bed. Attempt relaxation methods that might help you sleep. This will help your body to become rejuvenated in the morning. Try some visualizing and breathing techniques. Many people have a lot of luck with meditation, too.

161.   Keep a journal of everything that worries you. Allowing yourself to fixate on troublesome thoughts makes it nearly impossible to achieve peaceful sleep. Instead, write these problems and their solutions down so that you can put them in perspective. By getting a plan together, you can have less stress and sleep better in the night.

162.   Try doing some yoga or meditation before going to bed. Take your bath, get into something comfortable and then do your yoga or meditation. Both of these can help to clear your mind of stressful things and to relax your muscles so that you are able to fall asleep easier.

163.   Keep your bedroom at a cool temperature to give yourself the best chance for restful sleep. A drop in body temperature is an evolutionary signal for you to go to sleep. Try a warm bath before you turn in as well. The temperature of

your room should be about 65-70 degrees for optimal rest.

164.   Don't make yourself get in bed just because the clock on the wall says it is time. You'll sleep better if you wait until you're actually tired. That way, you can lay down, get comfy and drift off to sleep without worrying about how hard it is to do so.

165.   Many people have trouble falling asleep at night because of their mattress. We spend almost a third of our life on our mattress so it really needs to be comfortable. If it is too hard or soft, old or small, this could be the reason that someone suffers from insomnia.

166.   To get the best sleep your neck and spine should be aligned properly. They should form a straight line, not be bent or flexed. Your pillow may actually interfere with this position. It depends on your most comfortable sleep position. If so, try sleeping without a pillow at all or buying an orthopedic pillow.

167.   Deep breathing exercises are one of the most effective ways to combat insomnia. This exercise helps the brain release relaxing endorphins which help you drift off. Try inhaling slowly, holding

that breath for about three seconds, then letting it out slowly. Try this ten times. You should feel your body relaxing.

168.   Reduce carbohydrates in your meals during the day. Eating too many carbs at midday may result in feeling sluggish during the afternoon and getting your second wind late in the day, and this can prevent you going to sleep.

169.   A great technique to fall asleep is to practice deep breathing exercises when you can't fall asleep. Lie on your back then let your body relax. Hold each deep breath in your lungs for about three seconds, then exhale slowly. If you repeat this for around 5 minutes, you will feel increased relaxation, and are more likely to fall asleep.

170.   A good tip to use if you're dealing with insomnia is to take a warm bath. Taking a warm bath will relax you quite a lot, and will make it much easier for you to fall asleep. Be careful not to stay in too long though or you'll get fatigued.

171.   Keep your bedroom clean and free from clutter. Remove your television, computer and other electronic devices. Do not study, watch TV or work in bed. Decorate your bedroom in soothing colors that help you feel relaxed and

keep decorative items to a minimum. Your bedroom should be a relaxing place where you go to sleep.

172.   The stress of everyday activities can be a major cause of insomnia. Take some time before you get into bed to release the worries and stressful thoughts of the day. Practice deep breathing exercises, clear your mind, and make a list of things you will do the next day to release all worries from your mind.

173.   Don't read right before going to bed. You may love the time you have right before bed to get a few chapters in, but really you are stimulating your body. If you're battling insomnia that's the last thing that you want to do. So keep the books out of the room.

174.   Some people struggle with getting to sleep due to RLS. This is a medical issue that causes discomfort in the legs, which affects a person's sleep. It leads to constant movement with the legs where you makes it very hard to keep still. Restless Leg Syndrome can cause insomnia.

175.   Women are more prone to insomnia than men, and menopause could be one of the reasons why. Fluctuating hormones and hot

flashes can keep a menopausal woman awake at night. If this is the case, talk to your doctor, and see if hormone replacement therapy might help you sleep better.

176.   Don't automatically reach for prescription medicine when you can't fall asleep, as this can quickly become a dangerous habit. Insomnia is often temporary or simply due to something stressful going on in your life. Try other things first, like warm milk or a bath, and make sure you get an okay from your doctor before trying the heavy stuff.

177.   Although warm milk can be helpful for people who are struggling to sleep, some people do not enjoy milk or simply cannot consume dairy products due to an allergy. As an alternative, try a nice cup of herbal tea. That tea is all natural, and it really does relax the entire body. To find the best tea for you, check out health food stores to find a tea that will fulfill your needs.

178.   If you have trouble falling asleep on a regular basis, try to boost your melatonin levels. Tart cherry juice has been found to have high levels of melatonin. This can be found in natural or health food stores. A small amount a half an

hour before bedtime can really help you fall asleep and stay asleep.

179.   Your body needs to wake at a consistent time each day. Most people sleep in whenever they can to catch up on the missed sleep during the week. If you constantly suffer from insomnia, train your body to wake up at a certain time each day and stick to it!

180.   It is important that you have a minimal amount of stress pressing on you before your bedtime. Try relaxation techniques to fall asleep sooner. To get a good night of rest, both your body and mind should be relaxed. Meditation, imagery, and deep breathing exercises can help.

181.   The average mattress is only good for 8 years. After that time, your mattress may be lumpy or not giving you the support you need. Even if it seems OK, it may be a haven for dust mites and dead skin cells. This could also cause an allergic reaction which can keep you from sleeping well.

182.   Block out noise with white noise or earplugs. If you live in a busy area where you can't have a quiet night of sleep, take some measures to make your immediate environment quiet. You might

be able to try headphones that block out noise, earplugs, or white noise machines to block out other distracting noises.

183.   If you have trouble falling asleep at night, try keeping yourself on a regular sleep schedule. A regular sleep schedule is crucial if you are having trouble falling asleep. When you go to bed at about the same time on a daily basis, your body will be programed to sleep better and fall asleep quicker.

184.   Spend time each day exercising. Aerobic exercising should be done no less than 4 hours before your bedtime. If you wait until closer to your bedtime, you may cause more difficulty when trying to fall asleep. Early exercise can help to tire you out physically and make it easier for you to sleep when the time comes.

185.   If you find you wake up short of breath or in a panic, talk to your doctor about attending a sleep clinic. It is possible that you have sleep apnea, a condition where your airflow is cut off during the night. There are simple solutions for this condition which can give you the sleep you deserve.

186.   To sleep well, you must sleep comfortably. Invest in a good set of sheets, a high quality mattress and a reputable pillow. If your body can become completely comfortable while being supported totally, you will find that nothing is nagging at you, like a too-tight waistband on your pajama bottoms.

187.   Make sure that you consume Vitamin B during the day to aid with your sleep. This vitamin will help you have extra energy throughout the day so that you can stay as active as possible. This will make it easier to go to sleep as you will lack vitality before bedtime.

188.   The stress of everyday activities can be a major cause of insomnia. Take some time before you get into bed to release the worries and stressful thoughts of the day. Practice deep breathing exercises, clear your mind, and make a list of things you will do the next day to release all worries from your mind.

189.   Point your body from north to south. Put your feet towards the south and your head to the north. This actually aligns your body with the planet's magnetic field, essentially putting you in more harmony with the Earth itself. It may sound weird, but it works for many.

190.   Practice deep breathing when trying to sleep. This can relax your whole body. This can help you finally find that sleep you want. Breathe long inhales and exhales, repeatedly. Inhale through the nose and exhale through your mouth. Before you know it, you will feel your body begin to settle down.

191.   Adding a hot water bottle to your bed space may help you rest. The heat helps your body relax. That may be all that you need to cure your insomnia. One thing you can do is put a hot water bottle on your tummy. Breathe deep and relax. The heat will help you.

192.   Snoring, either your own or your partner's, can be a major cause of insomnia. To promote a restful night's sleep, speak with your doctor to eliminate the cause of your snoring. Keeping your bedroom properly humidified can ease congestion in nasal passages and reduce the snoring that keeps you from sleeping.

193.   Avoid sleeping on your side. To get a good night's sleep, rest on your back instead. If you simply can't fall asleep that way, try going to bed on your right side. The left side should be

avoided as it causes your liver and lungs to push up on your heart.

194.   Get up after half an hour. If you can't sleep, don't lay there for hours and hours. Get up and move to a nearby chair and read a little or try an activity. Do a very lowkey set of activities for a little while, and when you feel sleep, try again.

195.   Think about the things that bother you as you toss and turn. Now do something about them before you go to bed. Block out annoying lights and noises. Set the temperature at a cooler setting so you aren't hot and kicking off covers.If you eliminate the things that keep you awake, then sleep should come much easier.

196.   Remember reading bedtime stories as a child? This can work for grownups, as well. Try picking up an audio-book and letting it play as you are relaxing and getting ready to sleep. Low, soft music is also effective.

197.   If you are easily distracted by outside sounds, try using a white noise machine for sleep. Most people live in areas with various sounds art night, like traffic, barking dogs or neighbors talking. White noise machines are designed to drown out

this noise with a more relaxing sound, like rustling leaves or the sound of a waterfall.

198.   Sometimes when you have a hard time sleeping it is because your bed is not comfortable or a good fit for your body. Firm mattresses are good for those who have a hard time sleeping. If you can, invest in a good, firm mattress and you may find that you have an easier time with sleep.

199.   Try to keep things that are distracting out of the bedroom area. This only makes it more difficult for you to get to sleep. This means that computers, televisions and other electronics should not be in there. If they must be there, turn them off as soon as you are ready to hit the sheets.

200.   Caffeine may give you an instant pick me up in the morning, but keep in mind that high can last as long as 12 hours! That means you shouldn't have any caffeine after noon, and limit how much you get in the morning as well. Drink no more than two sodas, teas or coffees.

201.   Many people drink alcohol a little while before bed because it has been known to make them a little drowsy. While this may be true, drinking alcohol also increases the chances of

you waking up several times over the course of the night without being able to fall back asleep.

202.   While it is perfectly okay to use a sleep aid to help you rest every once in a while, this should not be used as a long-term treatment for insomnia. If you have been having sleepless nights for more than a week, it would be a good idea for you to see a doctor so he can properly diagnose and treat you.

203.   Try aromatherapy to help relax your mind and sooth your nerves. You can use a calming lavender bubble bath to relax in the tub. You might find that using a lavender scented laundry softener on your sheets works well too. Vanilla is also relaxing so consider using vanilla if you don't like lavender.

204.   To help fight insomnia, establish a regular sleeping schedule. If you regularly go to bed at the same time, your body gets used to that rhythm. As a result, you do not have to surprise your body with a new sleep schedule each day. Soon, your body will expect sleep at that given time.

205.   Try deep rhythmic breathing to snap out of a bout with insomnia. Lay in bed with your eyes

closed and simply breathe with deliberation. This exercise will relax you and help take the focus off of the price you will pay tomorrow for not getting enough sleep tonight. Try counting the breaths too, to get sleepy faster.

206.   If you find yourself having trouble with insomnia every night, stop drinking anything with caffeine in it by noon. This may sound extreme or like self-deprivation, but the effects of caffeine can actually be felt many hours after consumption. Enjoy your coffee or tea by lunch, and forgo them in the afternoon or early evening.

207.   Remember that caffeine isn't only found in coffee! Tea, pop and even chocolate all contain caffeine, as do energy drinks. You want to limit all the caffeine in your diet after 12pm so that you are able to fall asleep at night without the stimulating effects of this ingredient.

208.   If your insomnia is very severe, talk to your doctor about prescription sleep medications. While these medications are useful in treating insomnia, they are not to be taken on a long-term basis, as they can aggravate insomnia in the long run. They are best used in order to establish a sleep routine, and are then discontinued.

209.   Think of something pleasant. You might have a lot of random images passing through in your brain, but take control of those. Start visualizing very peaceful places. You can even count fuzzy sheep if you want. The most important thing is that you are encouraging your brain to think about something that may relax you.

210.   Set a wake up time and stick with it. If you get up for work at the same time each weekday, get up around that same time on the weekends. The more consistency you have in your sleep schedule, the better your body will adjust. You have to train your body to battle insomnia.

211.   Cherry juice may help you sleep. Studies have shown that drinking two glasses a day can help you sleep better than not drinking it at all. You will get great results if you drink tart juices.

212.   Learn stress busting remedies. If you don't address it, that stress is going to overwhelm you in the evening. Try deep breathing when you first tuck in, or yoga right before you retire, to alleviate the stress and be able to sleep.

213.   Exercise during the day. Exercise is a great way to get your body into shape, but it is also good for exhausting your body. A tired body has an easier time falling asleep at night. Aim for at least half an hour of exercise each day. Just be careful not to exercise too close to bedtime.

214.   Use your bed for sleep and don't use it as a place for activities like watching television. Don't take your laptop to bed, and use it to finish work. You want the bed to be a relaxing place. You don't want it mentally tied to stressful activities that don't involve rest or love.

215.   A good tip to consider if you've been suffering from insomnia is to see a doctor. Insomnia can be part of a larger problem, so you want to consult with a doctor to find out what exactly is causing the insomnia. Knowing what's causing it will make it easier to treat.

216.   Try your best to relax and keep stressful things out of your mind when bedtime is approaching. Have a cup of herbal tea and do something relaxing like listening to soft music or quietly reading a book. This will get you more in the move for sleep once your bedtime comes.

217.   If you are struggling with insomnia, try making yourself more comfortable! Studies show that when you are more at peace in the room, such as when lighting and sound are adjusted, you will sleep better and sleep longer. Move your furniture around, hang new curtains and invest in quality bedding to kick insomnia to the curb.

218.   Taking a nice warm bath can be extremely beneficial to helping you fall asleep. However, you never want to take too long of a bath because this is exhausting for your body. While you may think that it will help you even more to go to sleep, it will actually do the opposite.

219.   Warm milk is known to help relax you before bedtime. To warm the milk, place 8 ounces of milk in a small saucepan. Turn your stove on a medium low setting and slowly heat the milk up to 100 degrees. Avoid allowing the milk to boil because it may curdle.

220.   Chamomile is something that you can insert into your tea to help relax your body and the muscles that could be impacting your sleep. This herb is very relaxing and comes in natural form, offering many benefits and few side effects after consumption. Chamomile can be found in a local pharmacy or supermarket.

221.   Try your best to keep all of your work related tasks at the office and use your home as a sanctuary for relaxation. If there is something that must be done before you can start work the following day, you should try to arrive at the office a little early.

222.   To help fight insomnia, establish a regular sleeping schedule. If you regularly go to bed at the same time, your body gets used to that rhythm. As a result, you do not have to surprise your body with a new sleep schedule each day. Soon, your body will expect sleep at that given time.

223.   Try to set your alarm an hour earlier if you struggle with insomnia. While this may leave you feeling groggy for the morning, it should help you when you need to fall asleep later that night. Get up an hour earlier to prepare yourself for better sleep, later.

224.   Don't read right before going to bed. You may love the time you have right before bed to get a few chapters in, but really you are stimulating your body. If you're battling insomnia that's the last thing that you want to do. So keep the books out of the room.

225.   If you are having trouble sleeping, the first thing you should do is to visit your primary care physician. Occasionally, there is an underlying medical disorder that may be causing your symptoms. This could be as simple as stress or anxiety. However, it is best to be checked out and then go from there.

226.   Magnesium can help you fall asleep better. Magnesium can allow for more restful sleep. Magnesium rich foods include greens, pumpkin seeds and certain kinds of fish. Magnesium can also assist with the treatment of muscle cramps.

227.   Get your mind and body ready for sleep in advance. Dim the lights up to two hours before turning in. Practice meditation and void any activity that will make you think too much. Do some stretching exercises but nothing to strenuous. Relax with a cup of hot milk or non-caffeinated tea.

228.   Avoid participating in strenuous physical activity immediately before your bedtime. Because exercise causes your body to become excited. If you have problems sleeping, it is best to avoid exercising for several hours before you go to bed. Calming your body and mind prior to

bedtime boosts your chances of sleeping well at night.

229. Talk to friends and family about what worked for them. If you want to solve your insomnia problem, it might help to chat with people close to you to find out what works. You might also be able to get some support, so that they know that you are dealing with something.

230. Listen to music as you fall asleep. You can either look for music that you find soothing or you can use CDs that are made to help people fall asleep. CDs are available in steady patterns, soothing music or with words that can help you as you drift off to sleep.

231. If you suffer from insomnia, be sure you take the proper time to wind down before going to bed. It is easy to think that you could just go straight to bed after being on the go all day. Your body needs time to slow down a bit and relax before you actually put your head down on the pillow.

232. Have a sleep study done. If you are not able to sleep, or feel that you are having trouble staying asleep, you might have some form of sleep apnea that makes you unable to sleep

properly. A sleep study is the best way for people to determine this and find out what is going on.

233.   Don't use you bed for anything but sleeping. That means don't watch television in bed or bring work to do while in bed. It's best to not even have a television in your bedroom. Reading a relaxing book is probably fine or listening to soothing music. Consider your room as a relaxing refuge from the world.

234.   If you aren't able to sleep more than a few hours at night, then restrict yourself to only those hours in bed. For example, if you are sleeping 3 hours a night, then stay in bed for no longer than 3 hours. Once you start falling asleep immediately, increase it by an hour at a time. Be sure not to nap during the day as you try to fix your schedule.

235.   A bedtime snack that is high in carbs can help if you find it difficult to get to sleep. The reason to do this is because the snack will raise your blood sugar quickly, but the quick fall thereafter should help you relax into sleep.

236.   If you are one of the many people who can't fall asleep due to excess noise such as chirping crickets, or pattering rain, wear ear plugs. If you

don't want to use ear plugs, sleep with a small pillow covering your ear. Make sure you rotate the pillow as you flip to block out the noise.

237.   A warm bath will help to relax your body and lead you to a slumbering state. Upon getting out of the bath, you will have a lower body temperature, which often leads to sleep. Crawling happily into your bed after a nice warm shower or bath should lead to easy sleep.

238.   A good tip to consider if you've been suffering from insomnia is to see a doctor. Insomnia can be part of a larger problem, so you want to consult with a doctor to find out what exactly is causing the insomnia. Knowing what's causing it will make it easier to treat.

239.   Join an online forum for people who have insomnia. This way, you can interact with others who have the same problem you have. You can trade remedies that work, and you might be able to have a chat together if people are having a hard time sleeping. It's much easier to go through something if you aren't handling it alone.

240.   If you are struggling with insomnia, try making yourself more comfortable! Studies show

that when you are more at peace in the room, such as when lighting and sound are adjusted, you will sleep better and sleep longer. Move your furniture around, hang new curtains and invest in quality bedding to kick insomnia to the curb.

241.	Taking Melatonin may help you get you back to sleep. Melatonin is a naturally occurring hormone that is available in a supplement form. This hormone helps regulate the human sleep-wake cycle (circadian rhythm), causes drowsiness and lowers body temperature. Man-made Melatonin supplements are available at many health food and drug stores.

242.	Try imagining that it's the time to get up in the morning. This is sort of a fake out tip. You are trying to fake out your body to thinking it wants just a few more minutes rest, just like it does when that alarm goes off first thing in the morning.

243.	If you have trouble falling asleep on a regular basis, try to boost your melatonin levels. Tart cherry juice has been found to have high levels of melatonin. This can be found in natural or health food stores. A small amount a half an hour before bedtime can really help you fall asleep and stay asleep.

244.   Avoid sleeping on your side. To get a good night's sleep, rest on your back instead. If you simply can't fall asleep that way, try going to bed on your right side. The left side should be avoided as it causes your liver and lungs to push up on your heart.

245.   One thing that that you need to cut out of your life if you have trouble falling asleep is caffeine. The half-life of a dose of caffeine is about 7 hours. So if you drink a cup of coffee at 4pm, you will still have half of the caffeine racing through your body at 11pm. For restful and sound sleep, cut the caffeine out of your life.

246.   Examine your bed. Are your sheets nice to lay in? Are your pillows comfy and supportive? Is your mattress aged and sagging? It might be time to get a new bed or mattress. This can help allow you to relax and able to sleep.

247.   Sleep aids are truly addictive. It is wiser to speak with your physician as he may be able to provide alternatives for you.

248.   Your bed can become your friend when it comes to sleep if you make it exclusive to your sleeping time. Watching television throughout

the day, getting on the laptop, napping and other activities should be kept out of your bed. Your bed needs to only be used for sleeping only!

249.   If you are tired during the day, avoid taking a nap since this will increase your chances of staying awake far past your bed time. If you feel tired, take a shower, go for a jog or do anything else you can think of to stay awake until a little later.

250.   Some people have trouble getting to sleep and experience insomnia due to even the lightest of sounds. Therefore, many people have found it easier to sleep when they have earplugs in their ears. Wearing them blocks out any stray sounds, and you are able to better focus on clearing your thoughts and getting to sleep.

251.   Create ideal conditions in your room for sleep. That means making sure the temperature is on the right setting. Use a humidifier or an air purifier if needed. Eliminate annoying noises or bright lights. By creating a soothing atmosphere in your room, you will be able to fall asleep more easily.

252.   Try not to smoke any cigarettes or use any other products that contain nicotine too close to

bedtime. Many people get an endorphin rush when the nicotine hits their blood stream. This is not what you want to happen to you while you are struggling to get a little shut-eye.

253.   The darker your room, the better. It is shown the electronics can give off frequencies, both in light and sound, which can keep you awake at night. Take your cell phone, iPad and other devices to another room at night to help reduce the light and electronic noise in the room.

254.   If you were told to drink a warm glass of milk before bed to help you sleep, that advice was sound. This can help you feel drowsy and full, allowing you to pass right out. If you want an extra boost of sedation, add 1 tablespoon of honey to the mix.

255.   Create a set sleeping schedule. If you tend to go to sleep at random times it can cause a total nightmare for your internal clock. This can lead to serious insomnia over time. It's better to set a time every night that you go to sleep and a time that you wake up every day. Your body will respond to it quite well.

256.   Sleep as long as you can. Too many people with insomnia try to make themselves sleep as

long as possible. This usually backfires on them. They end up not getting any sleep or getting restless sleep. Just sleep as long as you naturally can to wake up feeling refreshed and rejuvenated.

257.   Don't be pessimistic. Don't keep saying that you have insomnia, and don't think you will have it forever. Positivity and a good mental state will be more conducive to sleep than constant complaints and fear will. Insomnia won't last your entire life, so rememeber that and know you'll get through it.

258.   Make sure that you consume at least eight glasses of water a day before you go to bed to help with your insomnia. Water helps to flush out the toxins from your body and can reduce the heavy feeling that you have when going to bed. Drink a glass right before bed to give your body the hydration that it needs to sleep.

259.   Set your alarm for an hour earlier than normal. You'll be tired in the morning, of course, but you'll probably feel sleepy that night. Get up an hour earlier to prepare yourself for better sleep, later.

260.　When insomnia is the enemy, reserve the use of your bed for sleep only. Sleep experts say that using your bed for reading, writing or watching TV will devalue it as a sleep aid. If your mind sees your bed as a place for sleeping only, your body will be conditioned to fall asleep faster.

261.　You can invite sleep in by creating a dark, soothing atmosphere in your bedroom. Be sure to get shades or curtains that block any outside light. Try some soothing music, or a CD with ocean or bird sound effects. Read a relaxing book. Find what works for you, and create a habit of it. You will learn to associate these activities with sleep.

262.　Some sunshine during the day can help you get to sleep during the night. Eat lunch outside or take a walk in the evenings. This helps your body produce melatonin to help you sleep easier.

263.　Be more proactive about the stress in your life, if you suffer with chronic insomnia. Stress is a leading cause of insomnia, so start eliminating the sources whenever possible, and do things for yourself that alleviate stress. Meditation or yoga can help, as can other forms of regular exercise. The less you stress, the more you sleep.

264.   Try a little house cleaning when your insomnia is getting the better of you. Many people find that being productive with a non-stressful task can help them reach a state that is more conducive to sleeping. Sweep the floor or dust your collectibles until you are more relaxed and feel completely tired.

265.   To avoid insomnia problems, remember not to drink beverages within the 3 hours preceding your bed time. You must make sure you get fluids during the day, but you don't want to fill up your bladder before bed. Getting interrupted by this when you're sleeping can really aggravate your insomnia, which is why it's not a good idea to drink anything a couple of hours before bed.

266.   You should write your issues in a sleep diary. Take notes of what foods you are eating, how often you work out and other habits. Then look at the amount of rest you are getting. When you understand the factors that get you less rest or more, you can make the changes you need.

267.   Get enough exercise. Exercise can help you cut stress by releasing endorphins into your system. That can help you sleep more deeply at night. However, avoid exercise within 3 or 4 hours before bed, because endorphins can keep

you awake if you exercise too close to your bedtime. Give it time.

268.   Remember that caffeine isn't only found in coffee! Tea, pop and even chocolate all contain caffeine, as do energy drinks. You want to limit all the caffeine in your diet after 12pm so that you are able to fall asleep at night without the stimulating effects of this ingredient.

269.   Your bedroom should be an environment that is designed for restful sleep. It needs to be dark, quiet and comfortable. Keep it at a temperature that is not too cold or too hot. When you combine all these things together, your bedroom will be the perfect environment to sleep in and you will not have trouble falling asleep.

270.   Human beings are evolved to see light as a signal to be awake. Try to keep light from interfering with your sleep, even small sources of light. Point your digital clock away from your eyes, as well as your cell phone or other small devices. These can hit your eyelids while you sleep, waking you up instinctually.

271.   Naps are the enemy of the insomniac. True, the appeal of a nap is hard to deny. A nap can be

enjoyable. This can make it hard for many people to rest during the night. While naps can give you more energy, they can give you too much and keep you awake at night.

272.   Many people suffer from insomnia because they cannot get their brain to shut down at night. One way to eliminate this is to write down any worries or problems before you go to bed. This will help your brain relax. When you make a list of your problems to be handled the next day, your brain can focus on what it needs to be doing, sleeping.

273.   Wear earplugs or purchase a white noise machine to block out all sounds while you are trying to get to sleep. Even if you don't think that small noises have a profound effect on your sleep patterns, there is a chance that this is what has been keeping you from getting your rest.

274.   Try aromatherapy to help relax your mind and sooth your nerves. You can use a calming lavender bubble bath to relax in the tub. You might find that using a lavender scented laundry softener on your sheets works well too. Vanilla is also relaxing so consider using vanilla if you don't like lavender.

275.   Research shows that getting plenty of natural light during the day helps you sleep better at night. Instead of staying in the office at lunch, eat outside. Don't wear sunglasses. Keep the windows open in your office, letting the light hit your face. You can even buy a light box if you live in a place that gets little light in the winter.

276.   Keep your bedroom clean and free from clutter. Remove your television, computer and other electronic devices. Do not study, watch TV or work in bed. Decorate your bedroom in soothing colors that help you feel relaxed and keep decorative items to a minimum. Your bedroom should be a relaxing place where you go to sleep.

277.   Many people swear by cookies and milk to gear up for a good night's sleep. The idea is that the carbs in the cookies, and the L Tryptophan in the milk induce sleepiness. Give it a try. The worst that can happen is that you get to eat cookies and milk at bedtime!

278.   Some people believe that carbohydrates can help you to fall asleep. A common suggestion is to eat a slice or two of white bread before bed with a cup of herbal tea. The carbs in the bread cause a tired, sluggish feeling that is conducive to

sleep, and the tea is relaxing, a good combination.

279.   Don't get too much sleep. If you cannot get to sleep after 30 minutes of lying in bed, try some relaxation or a soothing warm non-alcoholic beverage. Avoid taking naps during the day. If you must take a nap, keep it short and make sure it ends at least six hours before your normal bedtime.

280.   If insomnia is creeping up on you every night, consider getting earplugs. Many people are sensitive to sound, and don't even know it. Even quiet sounds will instigate insomnia, preventing needed rest. The earplugs will block out all sounds, and should help you get to sleep faster and stay asleep too.

281.   Ask your partner to give you a massage just prior to bed time. Even something as simple as rubbing your shoulders for a few minutes can help. Make sure they apply gentle, firm pressure to your body to help get rid of the tension in your muscles. This should make it much easier for you to sleep.

282.   If you have trouble falling asleep on a regular basis, try to boost your melatonin levels. Tart

cherry juice has been found to have high levels of melatonin. This can be found in natural or health food stores. A small amount a half an hour before bedtime can really help you fall asleep and stay asleep.

283.   Get up after half an hour. If you can't sleep, don't lay there for hours and hours. Get up and move to a nearby chair and read a little or try an activity. Do a very lowkey set of activities for a little while, and when you feel sleep, try again.

284.   Particularly if you work in an office and do not engage in much physical activity during the day, establish a workout schedule for yourself. Just 15 minutes a day of activity can help, as long as you do so a good 30 minutes or more before bed. Exercise enables you to get the oxygen you need to rest and sleep well.

285.   There is a direct link between exercise and better sleep. But be careful about exercising at night as it acts as a stimulant. Be sure that you're done with exercising about 3 hours before you go to bed so it doesn't make you have a hard time sleeping.

286.   Do you suffer from insomnia? Try taking a nice warm bath before you go to bed. This will

relax your muscles and reduce stress so that you can fall asleep when you go to bed. You need to make sure that it is a warm bath, not a hot bath. A hot bath can actually stimulate your body and prevent you from falling asleep.

287.   If you are getting up many times during the night to use the bathroom, your problem likely lies with your evening beverages. To stop this vicious cycle, quit drinking two hours before you go to bed. If you find that your thirst is voracious, talk to your doctor as you may have a medical issue at play.

288.   If you have a willing spouse, or sleep partner, try talking him or her into giving you a relaxing massage to help combat insomnia. If you cannot coerce them into a full-body massage, even a quick back massage with some soothing oil might be enough to relax your body, making sleep come easier.

289.   If your partner's snoring is keeping you up at night, get them to the doctor. Sleep apnea can cause your loved one to sputter and snore all night long, meaning you're not the only one who wakes up feeling lethargic! Apnea can lead to major health issues, so get their problem diagnosed as soon as possible.

290.   Just because it is time for bed doesn't mean you should try to sleep. Once you feel tired, then it is time to head on to bed. If you hold off until you're feeling tired, you'll be ready to fall directly off to sleep instead of obsessing over whether or not you'll have another bout of insomnia.

291.   Insomnia definitely has a negative impact on your life. Creating a firm sleep schedule is one way to keep yourself in line. By setting a fixed bedtime and waking hour, you train your body to adopt your routine. This applies to both your weekdays and weekends. Always rise at the appropriate time, even if you are fatigued. This can help you reprogram your body into a good sleep schedule.

292.   Some folks who are dealing with insomnia can actually trick their mind towards sleep. This is done by trying to imagine the feeling of having to get up. Some people keep visualizing their alarm ringing or themselves getting ready for work. If you can trick your mind into mentally clicking off the alarm, you might fall asleep easier.

293.   About three hours before bedtime, avoid all stimulants, such as caffeine, tobacco, alcohol and

certain medications. Caffeine effects can last for up to six hours, and alcohol, while sedating at first, can cause frequent wakefulness. Certain medications, such as for asthma, are stimulants as well. Check with your doctor to see if you can substitute, or make a different schedule.

294.   You need to sleep enough so that you have a sense of being rested. Remember that you cannot make up for lost sleep or get extra sleep in advance of challenges. Sleep only until you feel rested and do this on a regular basis. Don't "bank" hours one night and then cut back on others.

295.   Ask your partner to give you a massage just prior to bed time. Even something as simple as rubbing your shoulders for a few minutes can help. Make sure they apply gentle, firm pressure to your body to help get rid of the tension in your muscles. This should make it much easier for you to sleep.

296.   If you find you are troubled by insomnia, try to keep a journal of your thoughts before bedtime. Keep a note of all the things you do before heading off to bed. This might show a pattern of behavior that contributes to you having a bad night of sleep. It will be much

easier to take action against your insomnia when you know what's causing it.

297.   Many insomniacs lie in bed watching the minutes tick by on their clock. It can worry you to think about everything you have to do the next day. Don't stare at a clock. Turn it around or put it in another room so that it doesn't bother you.

298.   A relaxing massage prior to bed could be helpful in lessening the symptoms of insomnia. It works to relax the muscles and make the body feel calm. You and your spouse can alternate massages every night. There's no need for a full-body massage. Massaging the feet for 15 minutes works fine.

299.   It is likely that you already know that caffeine contributes to insomnia. There's no stimulant more popular than caffeine, because it does boost your metabolism. However, that also interferes a lot with sleep at night. You need to stop drinking caffeine pretty early. If you have nightly insomnia, stop consuming caffeine around 2pm.

300.   If you suffer from bouts of insomnia, take a look at your mattress to see if it may be

contributing to the problem. If your mattress is to soft, too hard, or just old and uncomfortable, it could be the cause of insomnia, or frequent night waking. A new mattress might be just what you need.

301.   Try to keep things that are distracting out of the bedroom area. This only makes it more difficult for you to get to sleep. This means that computers, televisions and other electronics should not be in there. If they must be there, turn them off as soon as you are ready to hit the sheets.

302.   Many people suffer from insomnia because they cannot get their brain to shut down at night. One way to eliminate this is to write down any worries or problems before you go to bed. This will help your brain relax. When you make a list of your problems to be handled the next day, your brain can focus on what it needs to be doing, sleeping.

303.   Smoking stimulates your body, so don't do it near bedtime. In fact, it's probably difficult for you to not smoke in the evening, so you are better off just to quit entirely. It will take a few months for your body to purge the toxins and

get back to normal, but it will leave you feeling amazing.

304.   Ask your partner if you snore. You may think you don't but your partner or friends know for sure. If you do snore, you may need to be checked for sleep apnea or congestion issues. Light snoring is usually treated with simple things such as choosing a position on your side to sleep in.

305.   To get the best sleep your neck and spine should be aligned properly. They should form a straight line, not be bent or flexed. Your pillow may actually interfere with this position. It depends on your most comfortable sleep position. If so, try sleeping without a pillow at all or buying an orthopedic pillow.

306.   Don't get too worked up about having insomnia. When you find yourself lying in bed again unable to sleep, it's easy to start getting frustrated and impatient. However, that behavior is not going to help usher in sleep. Try to realize that for many, insomnia can be fixed to some degree.

307.   For your afternoon snack, avoid eating foods which are processed. Instead, eat some fresh

fruit, yogurt or nuts. This will give you the energy boost you need without leaving you crashing or affected by high levels of sodium. Both situations can cause you to have trouble falling asleep at night.

308.   Have you checked your magnesium levels? Many people don't get enough magnesium in their diet, and taking a supplement can be a huge help. Commence a daily regime of taking these and see if a change occurs within the body. These pills can be found at reasonable prices at the local drug store.

309.   A bedtime snack that is high in carbs can help if you find it difficult to get to sleep. You may feel drowsy because of the rise and fall of your blood sugar levels.

310.   When insomnia becomes an obstacle to your being able to get adequate sleep, try increasing the ventilation in your bedroom. Doctors recommend this treatment for anyone having difficulty falling asleep, because improved breathing leads to a more relaxed state. Use a humidifier or open a window if you can, and finally get some rest.

311.   Exercise more to sleep better. Exercise will regulate hormones which will make it easier to sleep. Increase your exercise to balance your hormones and improve your sleep.

312.   You can invite sleep in by creating a dark, soothing atmosphere in your bedroom. Be sure to get shades or curtains that block any outside light. Try some soothing music, or a CD with ocean or bird sound effects. Read a relaxing book. Find what works for you, and create a habit of it. You will learn to associate these activities with sleep.

313.   Experts recommend making yourself more comfortable if insomnia is a problem for you. Change your bedroom around so that it is more conducive to sleep with light and sound. Add comfy pillows to your bedding ensemble, and make sure you don't wear anything constricting. The more comfortable you are, the more relaxed you will be, and that leads to better sleeping.

314.   Stop taking naps. If you take a nap during the day, you are going to have a harder time going to sleep and staying asleep at night. When you cut out your nap, you will find that you have a better time remaining asleep when you go to sleep for the night.

315.   Snoring, either your own or your partner's, can be a major cause of insomnia. To promote a restful night's sleep, speak with your doctor to eliminate the cause of your snoring. Keeping your bedroom properly humidified can ease congestion in nasal passages and reduce the snoring that keeps you from sleeping.

316.   Taking two tylenol when you go to sleep has always been a big tip for people with insomnia. However, you can trade this out with an ibuprofen. Or, you can substitute taking tylenol or ibuprofen with all-natural melatonin. All three of these are able to put you in a relaxed state.

317.   A massage before going to bed can be something that can keep insomnia at bay. A massage helps your body settle down for the night and eases tension from your muscles. Giving and getting massage are both relaxing, so be sure to trade off with your beloved so you can both sleep well. You don't have to do an intense full body massage, as 15 minute foot massages work well.

318.   Block out noise with white noise or earplugs. If you live in a busy area where you can't have a quiet night of sleep, take some measures to make

your immediate environment quiet. You might be able to try headphones that block out noise, earplugs, or white noise machines to block out other distracting noises.

319.	Keep your window open. Many people find that a bedroom filled with fresh air is conducive to better sleep. With an open window that allows the ambient temperature in your bedroom to be about 60 degrees Fahrenheit, you create the ideal environment for falling asleep. If you feel a bit chilly, simply add a blanket to your bed.

320.	It is as important that the things you sleep on are comfortable as it is that the room is dark and quiet. That means you need to have a quality mattress which is neither too hard nor too soft, a pillow which holds your head correctly, and night clothes which are loose and comfortable.

321.	Instead of letting your thoughts take control, put them down on paper. Better yet, write in your diary before bedtime and write down everything that has been bothering you throughout the day. Once you get these thoughts out of the system, you will go to sleep easier. Keep in mind that the point of this exercise is to avoid typing on a computer or any other electronic gadget that can keep you awake.

322.   Cherry juice may help you sleep. Studies have shown that people that consume cherry juice can go to sleep easier. You will get great results if you drink tart juices.

323.   If you are one of the many people who can't fall asleep due to excess noise such as chirping crickets, or pattering rain, wear ear plugs. If you don't want to use ear plugs, sleep with a small pillow covering your ear. Make sure you rotate the pillow as you flip to block out the noise.

324.   If you find that the fear of your alarm going off keeps you up, or causes you to awaken and not be able to fall asleep, consider buying a different alarm clock. There are clocks which use the gradual addition of light to the room which wake you calmly and leave you well rested.

325.   The effects of alcohol are funny as they can both sedate you and keep you up all night. While you may pass out quickly initially, you may also wake up feeling awful. On top of that, alcohol can cause you to become stimulated, totally reversing the sedative effects you felt at first.

326.   Many people find that soothing, quiet music can help them to fall asleep. First, it gives your

mind something to concentrate on which isn't nagging and is instead relaxing. Second, it covers up background noises which could disturb you, causing you to become stimulated and not be able to fall asleep.